This page intentionally left blank.

THE
TURMERIC
TESTAMENT:

*How This 4,000 Year-Old Golden Miracle
Naturally Fights Pain & Inflammation*

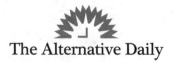

The Alternative Daily

This page intentionally left blank.

TABLE OF CONTENTS

Turmeric: trendy or true?

Health trends come and go; what was healthy for us a year ago has doctors up in arms today. However, that doesn't mean that all health trends are nothing more than celebrity endorsed fads. Turmeric is definitely having its moment in the health trend spotlight these days, leading many to ask the question: Is it just a trend or is there some truth to turmeric claims?

The Alternative Daily

Turmeric is topping food trend reports

A simple search on Pinterest (if you even have to search for it; chances are there's a suggested pin on the first page when you open the app) a quick Google search or even a query on WebMD will result in ample

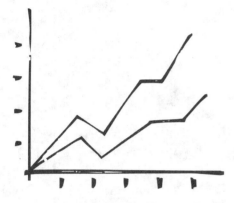

information about turmeric. These days, rice mixes, cold-pressed juices and teas infused with the bright yellow spice are a hit, causing the Sterling-Rice Group to declare turmeric as one of its Natural Nine 2015 Natural Food Trends.

This year, turmeric tops Google's list of food search trends, and it shows no sign of slowing down. One of the reasons is, as a whole, we're more interested in staying healthy and eating healthy. It turns out, we would rather add functional foods — like turmeric — to our meals than only focus on removing bad foods, and many agree that this is a healthier way of eating.

In the Think With Google report, 2016 Food Trends on Google: The Rise of Functional Foods author Pedro Pina notes, "Now, the focus of people's diets is less about eliminating foods than about adding them." Probiotics, coconut oil and a variety of spices top the

health-based searches via Google.
But according to Google's research
department, searches for turmeric
have grown 300 percent over the
last five years.

But it's not just our searches that
are exploding with the spice.
Beauty brands have jumped on the
turmeric bandwagon. Kiehl's has a
Turmeric & Cranberry Seed Energizing Radiance Masque. Companies
like Nestle are creating lines of "medical foods" that are supposed
to help treat diseases. It's clear that turmeric has joined the ranks of
apple cider vinegar, avocados and coconut oil as one of the functional
foods of which we can't get enough.

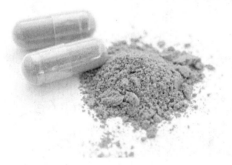

Turmeric has a long history in medicine

According to the National Institutes
of Health (NIH), turmeric has
been used in Vedic culture in India
for nearly 4,000 years. It was
traditionally used as a culinary
spice, but also held some religious significance. The NIH estimates that
by 700 A.D. turmeric could be found in China. By 800 A.D. it was in
East Africa, traveling to West Africa by 1200 A.D., and then to Jamaica

---

by the 1700s. According to ancient texts of the Ayurvedic and Unani systems, turmeric has been used for medicinal purposes in South Asia for centuries.

Turmeric's bright yellow color is thanks to a compound called curcumin, a natural anti-inflammatory agent. In fact, some studies have found that turmeric is as effective as over-the-counter anti-inflammatory drugs, just without the dangerous side effects. Studies and individuals claim that turmeric is effective for everything from the treatment of inflammatory bowel disease and rheumatoid arthritis to cancer prevention and lowering cholesterol.

So is turmeric a miracle root? Scientists are still studying its effects in a wide variety of conditions, but it's looking good for devotees of the spice. While researchers are 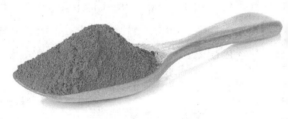 still discovering how turmeric may help us live better, it can't hurt to sprinkle it on fresh roasted vegetables or in your morning smoothie. It's sure to give any dish a flavor boost and it may just help you feel better in the long run.

One thing's for sure: if you haven't tried the spice, there's plenty of time. Its popularity means turmeric isn't going away any time soon.

What Is Turmeric?

Golden yellow in color, turmeric has a warm, bitter flavor that's also a little bit peppery. Its mild fragrance reminds you of ginger and Indian food — it's one of the primary spices in curry. It's also the ingredient that gives yellow mustard its vibrant color.

Where does it come from?

Turmeric was once called "Indian saffron" because its color resembled that of the coveted spice, but the two are in fact different spices. Saffron comes from the flower of the *Crocus sativus* and is native to Southwest Asia and Greece. Many describe saffron as having a floral, almost honey-like taste, giving it a flavor profile that's almost an exact opposite from that of turmeric.

Turmeric comes from the root of the *Curcuma longa*, an herbaceous plant that belongs to the ginger family, hence the similarities in fragrance. The *Curcuma longa* plant is native to the tropical regions of South Asia, specifically Indonesia and southern India. It needs a considerable amount of water to grow, and these regions are both the

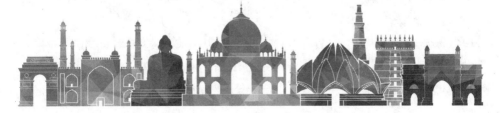

perfect temperature and humidity level for the plant to thrive. Nearly all of the globe's turmeric crop comes from India, and the country actually consumes about 80 percent of it, exporting the rest to other parts of the world.

According to the National Institutes of Health (NIH), the South Indian city of Erode — in the state of Tamil Nadu — is the world's largest producer of the spice. It's often referred to as "turmeric city" or the "yellow city."

How is it grown and harvested?

The plant is harvested for its rhizome (a long, continuous underground stem system that shoots roots out into the ground at intervals) and reseeded from some of those rhizomes for the following

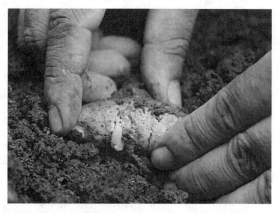

growing season. Once harvested, the turmeric rhizome of the *Curcuma longa* plant is dried and ground to a yellow powder — but it's not as easy as just pulling the root out of the ground and hanging it up to dry.

Traditionally, cow dung was used to help process turmeric. For hygienic reasons, the practice of placing rhizomes in earthenware with water and then covering it in leaves and a layer of manure has gone out of favor. These days, according to the NIH, rhizomes are placed in shallow pans of alkaline water and boiled for different lengths of time depending on the region and variety — 40 to 45 minutes in India, six hours in Pakistan — before they're dried in the sun. The boiling process helps to remove the strong, earthy odor from the raw root, and also serves to gelatinize the starch in the root and give the spice its uniform yellow color. In fact, that color will not fade over time, although sunlight and heat exposure will deplete the powdered spice of its flavor.

Purchasing and storing turmeric

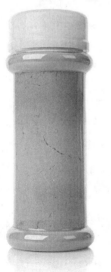

Although turmeric's growing popularity means that you can pick it up at many grocery stores, instead check out ethnic markets, organic grocery stores or local spice stores, where you may be able to pick up turmeric produced in smaller batches. Always go for organic, no matter where you acquire your turmeric. Be sure to store it in a cool, dry and dark place to ensure its flavor lasts as long as possible. If you choose to grate your own turmeric, the whole rhizome should be stored in the vegetable crisper of the refrigerator.

HISTORY OF TURMERIC

About the same time that
Stonehenge is believed to have been
completed, the Eleventh Dynasty
was coming to an end in Egypt,
and the Bronze Age had begun
in Ancient China, turmeric was
first being used for culinary and
religious reasons. Dating back 4,000
years, turmeric's use in Vedic culture in India has a long tradition. In
fact, archeologists have found residue from ginger, garlic and turmeric
in pots discovered near New Delhi dating back to 2500 BCE. As the
civilizations of the world began to become more aware of one another
and trade increased, turmeric traveled to other parts of the globe:
China, East Africa, West Africa and Jamaica.

By the eleventh century, the Western world had become aware of
the spice, thanks in larger part to Marco Polo. The merchant-traveler
mentioned turmeric in his writings while traveling in China, dated
1280 BCE. "There is also a vegetable that has all the properties of
true saffron, as well as the smell and the color, and yet it is not really
saffron." Turmeric soon became known throughout medieval Europe
as "Indian saffron," and was used as a far less expensive substitute for
the coveted spice.

However, according to Michael Castleman, author of The Healing Herbs: The Ultimate Guide to the Curative Power of Nature's Medicines, "The ancient Greeks were well aware of turmeric, but

unlike its close botanical relative, ginger, it never caught on in the West as either a culinary or medicinal herb. It was, however, used to make orange-yellow dyes. In the 1870s, chemists discovered turmeric's orange-yellow root powder turned reddish brown when exposed to alkaline chemicals. This discovery led to the development of turmeric paper... to test for alkalinity."

The many names of turmeric

In the east, however, turmeric was revered as a sacred and medicinally helpful spice. Its numerous names are an indication of the breadth of uses for the spice from thousands of years ago.

In the exhaustive volume, Herbal Medicine: Biomolecular and Clinical Aspects, Second Edition, authors Sahdeo Prasad and Bharat B. Aggarwal note that turmeric has been known by many different names throughout history. For example, it became known as "haldi" in North India, which comes from the Sanskrit word *haridra*. It was known as *terre merite* in French, which simply translates to "yellow root," but in comparison to the 53 different names for the spice in Sanskrit, the French equivalent seems lackluster.

Some of the Sanskrit names for turmeric are as follows:

- *Anestha:* not offered for sacrifice or homa
- *Bhadra:* auspicious or lucky
- *Haridra:* precious to hari, Lord Krishna
- *Hridayavilasini:* charming or delights the heart
- *Jayanti:* wins over diseases
- *Jawarantika:* one that cures fevers
- *Mehagni:* kills fat
- *Pavitra:* holy
- *Varavarnini:* gives one a fair complexion
- *Vishagni:* poison killer
- *Yoshitapriya:* beloved of the wife — presumably Parvati, wife of Lord Shiva

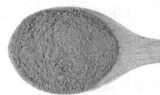

Many of turmeric's names describe its beauty, color or length, but others, like *jawarantika* above, indicate medicinal uses for the spice. Other names symbolize the beliefs that turmeric brings prosperity or helps you live free from desires.

Traditional medicinal uses for turmeric

In Ayurvedic medicine, turmeric is believed to treat many ailments and infuse overall strength to the body's energy. Other uses of turmeric in the Ayurvedic tradition include regulating menstruation, relieving arthritis, dissolving gallstones, ridding the body of worms and improving digestion. Today, Ayurvedic providers recommend turmeric for the treatment of respiratory conditions, anorexia, diabetic wounds, coughs, sprains, inflammation and liver conditions.

In South Asian countries, turmeric has long been used for its antibacterial properties and is often applied to cuts, bruises and

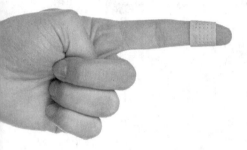

burns. Turmeric is used similarly in Pakistan and Afghanistan, where it is applied to a burnt cloth and then placed on a wound. The belief is that turmeric will keep the wound clean and speed up the patient's recovery.

Spiritual significance of turmeric

As some of the names for turmeric suggest, the spice also holds spiritual and religious significance. The Hindu religion, for example, has held turmeric as sacred and auspicious for centuries. According to PBS writer Tori Avey, Hindu weddings include a bright yellow string dyed with turmeric paste, which the groom ties around his new wife's neck. The string is known as the *mangala sutra*, a symbol that the woman is married and ready to run the household.

In other parts of India, a piece of the turmeric rhizome is sometimes worn as a protective amulet against evil spirits. Bright yellow Buddhist robes are often dyed in turmeric, and in the southwest Indian state of Kerala, children wear turmeric-dyed clothing during the Onam festival, as it is closely associated with Lord Krishna.

The West begins to be interested in turmeric

Research into turmeric began in Germany sometime in the early 1920s. According to Daniel B. Mowrey, "Sesquiterpenes in the essential oil of turmeric were isolated in 1926 and to them was ascribed the therapeutic activity," of the spice. Mowrey points out that numerous experiments were conducted on the spice and its essential oil. The results of these experiments found that turmeric might help stimulate bile flow in the body, helping with gallbladder conditions. Mowrey pointed out, "The flavonoids [of turmeric] cause the contraction of the gallbladder and thereby increase the effective emptying of this organ."

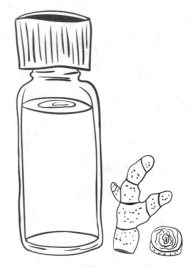

Western awareness of turmeric's effects began to spread further in the 1960s with the publication of Rudolf Weiss' Herbal Medicine in 1961. Although Weiss confirms that turmeric may help the gallbladder, he also cautions against its use, noting that the bright yellow color might be an irritant to the gastric system. He cites people's reactions to very spicy Indian curry as evidence, discounting the fact that there are more spices present in curry than just turmeric.

Interest in turmeric in the West didn't swell until the 1990s when herbalists began promoting its use. Today, there are thousands of studies focused on turmeric's medicinal value. In 2011, Herbal Medicine: Biomolecular and Clinical Aspects noted "over 3,000 publications dealing with turmeric that came out in the last 25 years."

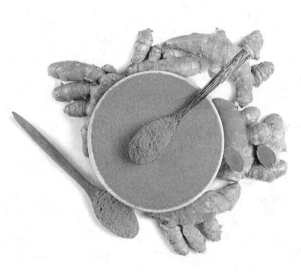

Turmeric is now lauded as a remedy for many ailments, for anything from skin conditions to reducing parasites. We now know what the ancients believed: turmeric might just be a miracle spice.

Nutritional profile

Turmeric offers a wide range of nutritional benefits, not the least of which is its curcumin content — the compound that gives turmeric its bright yellow color. Curcumin has been shown to reduce inflammation in the body, and there's some evidence that it might inhibit the growth of tumors. Combined with turmeric's other nutrients, the spice offers a wealth of nutritional benefits.

Turmeric is a good source of manganese and iron, and also contains vitamin B6, vitamin C, vitamin E, fiber, copper, niacin, zinc and potassium. In just two teaspoons of turmeric, you can consume 17 percent of your daily manganese needs, and 10 percent of your daily iron needs.

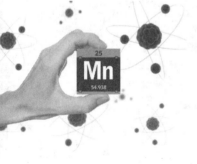

Manganese is an antioxidant that benefits mitochondria, the energy producing part of cells. According to Oregon State University's Linus Pauling Institute, "Because mitochondria consume over 90 percent of the oxygen used by cells, they are especially vulnerable to oxidative stress." Oxidative stress contributes to the breakdown of cell structures in the body, which is involved in the development of many conditions including Parkinson's and Alzheimer's disease, as well as infections, chronic fatigue syndrome and depression. Iron aids in metabolism, development and in the synthesis of some connective tissue and hormones.

Turmeric's recommended daily allowance and ORAC value

The recommended daily allowance for turmeric is 100 grams, and those 100 grams are full of amazing nutritional benefits including:

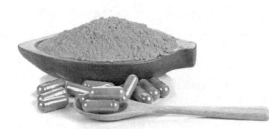

- 53 percent of your daily dietary fiber
- 138 percent vitamin B6
- 32 percent niacin
- 43 percent vitamin C
- 21 percent vitamin E
- 54 percent potassium
- 517 percent iron
- 340 percent manganese
- 40 percent zinc

Of course, these percentages are only accessible in supplement form, and you should always consult your healthcare provider before adding a supplement to your health regime. If it's right for you, turmeric's Oxygen Radical Absorbance Capacity (ORAC) value — the measurement of an antioxidant's capacities — is among the highest available, and a great addition to a healthy diet.

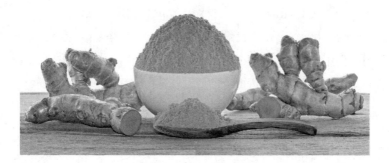

Medicinal Value of Turmeric

Still on the fence about turmeric or convinced it's a fad? There's a wealth of scientific evidence that supports claims that turmeric's healing properties — thanks to the active compound curcumin — are based in truth. From its anti-inflammatory properties to its ability to help reduce stress levels, turmeric has been shown to aid the body and mind in various ways.

Turmeric's antibiotic, antifungal, anti-inflammatory and antiviral properties

Antibiotic properties

The curcumin in turmeric was found to be an effective antibiotic in a study conducted by a team from Jawaharlal Nehru University in New Delhi and the India Beijing Institute of Microbiology and Epidemiology in 2015. Researchers tested the compound against four different bacteria types: *S. aureus, E. faecalis, E. coli,* and *P. aeruginosa.* They found that curcumin actually breaks down the membranes of these bacteria, causing them to essentially fall apart, thanks to a leaky membrane.

In another study, published in *FEMS Immunology and Medical Microbiology*, scientists found that curcumin "significantly inhibited" the *Vibrio vulnificus* infection, a bacterium from the same family as cholera. It is most often contracted when a person comes in contact with seawater or seafood, and causes gastrointestinal problems including diarrhea, vomiting and abdominal pain. Perhaps a sprinkling of turmeric on your oysters is a good idea!

Antifungal properties

People with compromised immune systems are more susceptible to fungal infections and we're learning more about them all the time. Candida has become a topic of much conversation lately, and with good reason. The fungal infection can cause fatigue, brain fog, hormone imbalance, a loss of sex drive, bad breath, digestive problems, urinary tract infections and many more ailments. However, a 2011 study from the Department of Biosciences at Jamia Millia Islamia in New Delhi, India, found that curcumin displayed antifungal properties when tested on 14 strains of candida.

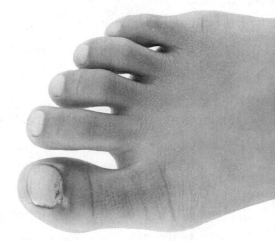

Turmeric may help treat other fungal infections as well. Individuals who suffer from chronic asthma can become infected with Oropharyngeal candidiasis (OPC). In fact, OPC is very common for people who have to undergo treatment for the condition. Curcumin's antifungal and anti-inflammatory properties we found to help reduce the fungal burden on chronic asthma sufferers in a 2011 study. It appears that turmeric is a must-have for anyone with asthma.

Anti-inflammatory properties

When a part of the body is injured, white blood cells and other protective substances flood to the area in an attempt to protect it from further injury or to fight infection. This process, in the short term, is natural and healthy. However, when chronic inflammation sets in, it might be a sign of an autoimmune disease.

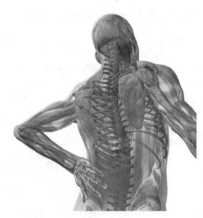

Naturopaths and other practitioners have long recommended that patients use turmeric for its anti-inflammatory properties.

One study investigated the effect of turmeric on the treatment of arthritis. The 2006 study from the University of Arizona found that turmeric reduces joint inflammation and joint destruction in live subjects, making it a viable treatment option for those who suffer from the condition.

In 2003, the University of California conducted a literature review on the anti-inflammatory uses of turmeric curcumin. The reviewer found that the traditional claims of turmeric's anti-inflammatory properties were valid— as well as the antioxidant, antiviral and antifungal properties. It also found that people who consume excessive amounts of the spice — 8,000 milligrams of curcumin per day for three months — did not experience any toxic effects as a result.

Antiviral properties

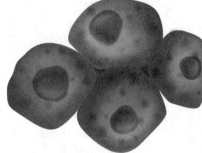

Many patients who have contracted the hepatitis C virus (HCV) undergo liver transplantation surgery. However, the reinfection of the graft is a very real health threat for these patients. In an attempt to find a natural and affordable antiviral agent, researchers tested human liver cells to learn if turmeric blocked HCV from entering new, uninfected cells. The 2014 study published in the medical journal *Gut* found that curcumin actually inhibits the entry of hepatitis C virus genotypes into human liver cells. The team also found that turmeric prevents the virus from binding with liver cells.

Another study found that a curcumin-based vaginal cream kills human papillomavirus (HPV) cells. The 2013 test-tube study found that curcumin prevented the expression and spread of pro-cancer proteins when introduced to HPV cells. HPV has been shown to cause cervical cancer.

CONDITIONS TURMERIC MAY HELP

Cancer

Research is still
developing on the role of
turmeric and curcumin in
the treatment of cancer. It
is generally recommended
that if you consume
turmeric as a cancer
patient, it should be done

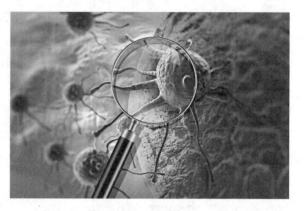

alongside mainstream treatments, as alternative therapies like herbal
supplements have not been shown to fight cancer alone. That said,
there's some evidence that turmeric may help prevent some cancers
— skin, colon, breast and prostate — and may help support cancer
patients through their treatment.

Multiple studies have shown that turmeric may help reduce pain and
lower signs of oxidative stress in patients undergoing chemotherapy
and other cancer treatments. In a review of nearly 3,000 studies by
The University of Texas MD Anderson Cancer Center, researchers
found that turmeric "affects numerous pathways linked with
tumorigenesis [the formation of tumors] and thus has potential both
for prevention and treatment of cancer."

Researchers note that the largest problem with curcumin supplementation is the limited bioavailability of the compound. The team notes that more clinical trials are needed "to fully appreciate its potential," but turmeric's relatively low cost and lack of side effects make it a worthy object of study in cancer treatment.

Another study published in the journal *Molecular Urology* found that turmeric may prevent prostate cancer, while another study published in the *Archives of Pharmacal Research* found that curcumin inhibits the growth of cancer cells in human breast tissue.

Cardiovascular disease and cholesterol

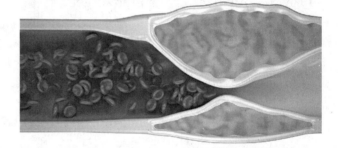

Cardiovascular disease is caused by the hardening and thickening of the arteries. It can cause heart attack and stroke, but turmeric may help prevent some of the life-threatening effects of the disease — and the disease itself.

Turmeric has a fascinating effect on cells, not the least of which is that it stops platelets in the blood from clumping together. This property means that turmeric may help prevent blood clots from building up along the walls of arteries.

In 2012, a study published in the *American Journal of Cardiology* found that turmeric extract might prevent heart attacks for patients who undergo bypass surgery. While the study is based on a relatively small sample set, the results are encouraging. In the study, 121 patients who underwent non-emergency bypass surgery between the years of 2009 and 2011 were either given a placebo or one gram of curcumin four times a day for three days before their surgery. The patients continued taking the capsules for five days post-surgery.

Only 13 percent of the patients who took curcumin before and after surgery experienced a heart attack, while 30 percent of the placebo group had a heart attack. That means that patients who took curcumin before and after their surgery had a 65 percent lower chance of heart attack than their counterparts.

As far back as the 1990s, researchers have investigated turmeric's ability to reduce LDL cholesterol levels. LDL cholesterol is considered the "bad" cholesterol. Small early studies found that turmeric's active compound, curcumin, lowers LDL cholesterol levels in human subjects. One such study found that just 500 milligrams of curcumin per day for a week lowered LDL cholesterol levels by 33 percent. The study also showed that their total cholesterol level dropped by nearly 12 percent, while their "good" HDL cholesterol levels increased by 29 percent.

Diabetes and blood sugar

Diabetes is a serious metabolic disease with potentially life-threatening complications. Patients with diabetes do not produce enough insulin, and so they experience elevated levels of glucose in the blood stream.

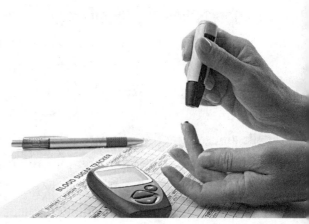

In a randomized, double-blind study published in the journal *Drugs in R&D*, 67 subjects were studied to see if 300 milligrams of curcumin 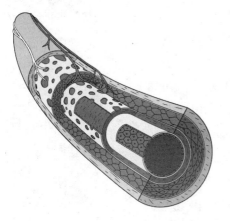 twice a day would help support the health of their endothelial function — the function of the inner lining of the blood vessels. Diabetic and hyperglycemic patients often experience oxidative stress that leads to dysfunction of this part of the circulatory system. According to the study, curcumin had a significant positive effect on subjects' blood vessel function. The effect was so significant, in fact, that it was comparable to the results experienced by the sample group who took atorvastatin, a statin prescribed to improve blood vessel health and lower cholesterol.

Supports healthy blood sugar

Curcumin may help prevent diabetes by helping to support healthy blood sugar levels. In a 2012 study published in the journal *Diabetes Care*, researchers studied the effects of nine months of curcumin treatment on pre-diabetic subjects. The randomized, double-blind, placebo-controlled study found that those who took curcumin supplements daily were significantly less likely to develop type 2 diabetes. The results of the study prompted the authors to conclude that curcumin intervention might be beneficial to pre-diabetic individuals in the regulation of their blood sugar and the prevention of disease.

Gastrointestinal conditions

There are many gastrointestinal conditions that turmeric may help. From improved digestion to the prevention of gas and bloating, turmeric supports a healthy digestive tract in many ways. However, doctors recommend you do not take turmeric or curcumin supplements if you have a stomach ulcer. According to the University of Maryland Medical Center, "Turmeric does not seem to help treat 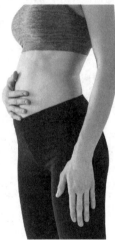 stomach ulcers. In fact, there is some evidence that it may increase stomach acid, making existing ulcers worse." As always, consult your healthcare provider before taking a new supplement.

Improves digestion

Sufferers of indigestion might be interested to know that curcumin may help soothe their digestive tract. Turmeric has a long tradition of being used to treat gallbladder issues, as it stimulates the organ to produce bile. After studying the spice, the German Commission E —the organization that determines which herbal remedies are medically safe — has approved turmeric for the treatment of digestive issues, including indigestion.

In a placebo study published in the *Journal of the Medical Association of Thailand*, turmeric supplements were found to be significantly effective in the treatment of indigestion. In the study, 116 adult subjects were split into three groups: 41 subjects in the placebo group, 36 in a group that received flatulence medication, and 39 who received curcumin supplements. At the end of the study, 53 percent of the placebo subjects reported improved digestion, while 83 percent of the flatulence medication group reported similar improvements. The curcumin supplement group, however, reported an 87 percent improvement in digestion and were not exposed to any potentially adverse side effects in the process.

Prevents gas and bloating

Abdominal gas and bloating are often caused by inflammation of one sort or another. Turmeric's anti-inflammatory and antioxidant properties make it useful for the treatment and prevention of gas and bloating. A German study conducted in 2010 found that two antioxidants, resveratrol and curcumin, as well as the medicine simvastatin, reduce inflammation in the digestive tract.

Researchers actually found that the three together "preserved intestinal barrier functions as indicated by reduced bacterial translocation rates in [the] spleen, liver, kidney and blood." Resveratrol is found in a number of foods, including pistachios, peanuts, red wine, blueberries, and dark chocolate. Maybe a blueberry and dark chocolate smoothie with turmeric sprinkled on top should be on your breakfast menu if you suffer from gas or bloating!

Reduces parasites

One of the many traditional uses of turmeric is the treatment of patients with parasitic infections. Such parasites might include tapeworms, roundworms or pinworms. These little bugs can cause nausea or vomiting, diarrhea, abdominal pain, gas, bloating, fatigue, weight loss or even dysentery.

However, there's good news for those living in areas where parasites are known to populate. In animal tests, infected subjects have experienced a significant reduction of parasites when given curcumin supplements. There are also a few studies that have found curcumin to be effective in the prevention of several kinds of parasites. The results were so profound as to suggest that turmeric may be a very effective chemopreventative measure against some really bad intestinal bugs.

Remission support for ulcerative colitis

Ulcerative colitis is a chronic disease of the digestive tract that, in severe cases, can cause life-threatening complications. But there's good news for those who have the disease. In a double-blind placebo-controlled study from the Hamamatsu University School of Medicine and the Hamamatsu South Hospital in Hamamatsu, Japan, subjects who had ulcerative colitis 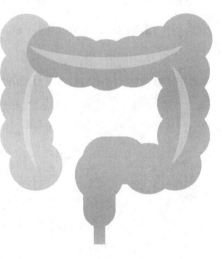 in remission and took curcumin experienced a significantly lower relapse rate than the control group. There is also some evidence that curcumin's anti-inflammatory and antioxidant properties may help those with inflammatory bowel diseases, like Crohn's disease.

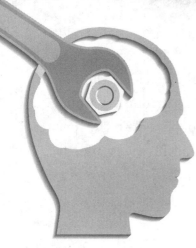

MENTAL SUPPORT

Animal studies have found that curcumin may provide antidepressant-like benefits for those who struggle with depression. The implications for human patients is incredible. Turmeric may also help boost your mood and combat PTSD.

Boosts mood

When combined with black pepper, turmeric may help you maintain a sunny outlook on life. In a 2008 study published in *Psychopharmacology*, researchers from India found that curcumin helps to boost the neurotransmitters responsible for happiness and reward — serotonin and dopamine — in animal subjects, especially when combined with piperine, the active ingredient in black pepper. Although there are no human trials at this time, the implication is that we may experience the mood enhancing benefits of turmeric when mixed with black pepper. If you're having a down day, it might be worth trying.

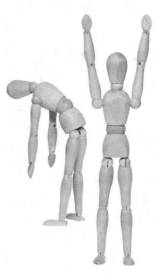

Combats depression

Turmeric may also help combat depression in those with major depressive disorder. In a 2014 study titled "Efficacy and safety of curcumin in major depressive disorder: a randomized controlled trial," researchers found that subjects who took a combination of curcumin supplements and fluoxetine — a medicine prescribed for depression and obsessive compulsive disorder, often under

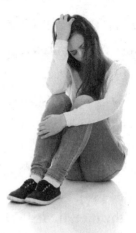

the generic name Prozac — experienced improved mental states. According to the authors, "This study provides first clinical evidence that curcumin may be used as an effective and safe modality for treatment in patients with MDD [major depressive disorder] without concurrent suicidal ideation or other psychotic disorders."

Eases PTSD Symptoms

Studying the effects of curcumin in Pavlovian fear memories "a widely studied animal model of traumatic memory formation in posttraumatic stress disorder (PTSD)," researchers from Hunter College, Yale, and The City University of New York found that curcumin might help inhibit new and reactivated fear memories in humans. According to the study, it appears that curcumin might be able to impair "fear memory consolidation and reconsolidation processes," making it a potentially beneficial treatment for those who suffer from PTSD.

Helps reduce stress

Stress contributes to a number of conditions and diseases like heart attack, stroke, depression, anxiety, gastrointestinal issues and more. However, turmeric may help reduce stress as part of a healthy diet. In a 2009 study, 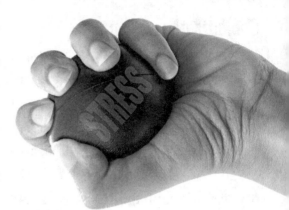 animal subjects experienced significantly reduced stress-induced behavior when they were undergoing curcumin treatments. They also showed significantly fewer biochemical and neurochemical reactions to stress when receiving curcumin supplements.

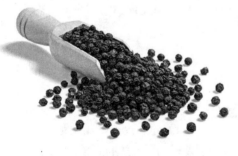 When curcumin was supplemented with piperine (or black pepper), which is a known bioavailability enhancer, subjects showed enhanced neurotransmitter processing. As a result, the authors noted, "This study provided a scientific rationale for the use of curcumin and its co-administration with piperine in the treatment of depressive disorders" as well as stress levels.

Neurodegenerative and autoimmune diseases of the brain

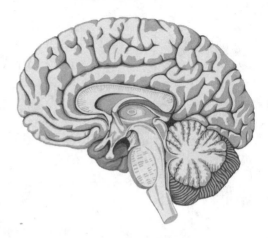

Turmeric is one of the foods that Dr. David Perlmutter recommends in his book, Brain Maker: The Power of Gut Microbes to Heal and Protect Your Brain – for Life. According to Dr. Perlmutter, turmeric stimulates the Nrf2 pathway. "When this is triggered," writes Dr. Perlmutter, "it causes the body to make higher levels of protective antioxidants, while reducing inflammation and enhancing detoxification." Oxidative stress and inflammation are two of the causes of neurodegenerative diseases, like Alzheimer's, Parkinson's and multiple sclerosis. If turmeric can in fact reduce oxidative stress and inflammation, it may be a very effective treatment for these diseases.

Prevents the progression of Alzheimer's disease

Alzheimer's disease is a progressive disease in which patients experience a growing decline in mental abilities. They eventually experience significant behavioral changes and a decline in their ability to complete everyday tasks. Many studies note that there is a significantly lower incidence and prevalence of Alzheimer's disease in India, where turmeric is consumed as part of a regular diet.

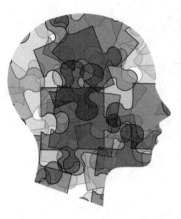

In a review of studies focused on turmeric's effects on Alzheimer's disease published in the *Annals of Indian Academy of Neurology*, the authors note that curcumin's anti-inflammatory and antioxidant properties have been shown to support brain health. "Based on the main findings," the authors note, "curcumin will lead to a promising treatment for Alzheimer's disease." Although more human trials are needed to determine the full extent of curcumin's effect on Alzheimer's patients, the research is promising.

Reduces the risk of Parkinson's disease

Turmeric's anti-inflammatory and antioxidant powers cannot be overstated. It is believed that free radicals and inflammation are among the primary causes of Parkinson's disease, but turmeric may counteract those. When patients are treated for Parkinson's disease, they are often prescribed medication or supplements that mimic dopamine.

Recent studies have shown that several spices may have this ability, including curcumin. Although further studies are needed to determine if turmeric may aid in the treatment and management of Parkinson's disease, its anti-inflammatory and antioxidant properties are certainly a help in the prevention of the degenerative disease.

Slows the progression of multiple sclerosis

Multiple sclerosis is an autoimmune disease, meaning that the immune system attacks a part of the body as if it were a foreign substance. In the case of multiple sclerosis, the brain and spinal cord suffer through damage to the myelin sheath, the protective cover surrounding neurons. When the myelin sheath breaks down, nerve cells cannot send signals to other cells as quickly or as effectively as healthy nerve cells. The most recognizable outward effect is patients' difficulty controlling their bodies.

In an animal study from 2008 that investigated a similar condition to multiple sclerosis,

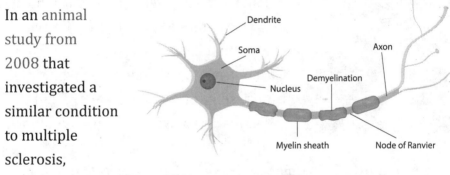

researchers found that the rats who received curcumin supplementation had a significantly less severe experience with the disease. The implication is that curcumin might be an effective treatment for humans with multiple sclerosis.

Many researchers have found that T cells — lymphocytes that are produced by the thymus gland and are active during the immune response — may play a role in preventing multiple sclerosis. The thought is that T cells are much lower when a patient with multiple sclerosis is experiencing an attack, so boosting the cells might prevent the progression of the disease. In a study titled, "Curcumin modulation of IFN-beta and IL-12 signaling and cytokine induction in human T cells," researchers found that curcumin helped stimulate T cells, adding more evidence to the claim that turmeric may help slow the progression of multiple sclerosis.

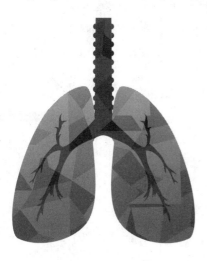

Respiratory support

Respiratory problems like asthma, bronchitis or COPD are caused by inflammation brought on by some kind of trigger, whether it's allergies or lifestyle choices that have damaged the respiratory tract. Turmeric may help those who suffer from respiratory issues, thanks to its anti-inflammatory powers. For instance, many people claim that turmeric helps with sinus issues. So, the next time you are suffering from a cold or nasal congestion, try turmeric powder in the warm milk of your choice. It might help clear those passages.

Helps quiet coughs

Coughs happen for a number of reasons, from allergies to illness. Although there have not been any studies looking specifically at turmeric's effect on coughs, one study investigated the effectiveness of honey and turmeric together as a cough treatment. The study was relatively small, but found that those who received 15 milliliters of honey and 200 milligrams of turmeric powder twice a day for three days experienced improved health and a reduced cough when compared to those who did not. Honey is known for its own antimicrobial properties, so it's not surprising that when the two are combined, the results are significant.

Improves asthma

Asthma sufferers experience a constriction of the airways, sometimes accompanied by spasms of the bronchial tubes in the lungs. They often are hypersensitive to allergens and can sometimes experience difficulty breathing. Several studies have shown that inhaling turmeric fumes can improve asthma by reducing airway inflammation.

Reduces the effects of COPD

Chronic obstructive pulmonary disease (COPD) is an inflammatory disease that affects the lung tissue, often due to extended exposure to cigarette smoke. There's a close link between COPD and lung cancer, making it even more worrisome, but it looks like turmeric may help those who suffer from COPD.

In a study titled, "Curcumin inhibits COPD-like airway inflammation and lung cancer progression in mice," the team or researchers found that curcumin significantly suppressed chemokines that are involved in the progression of lung cancer in COPD patients. They also found that curcumin reduced intrinsic and extrinsic inflammation that tends to lead to cancer.

Soothes bronchitis and other issues

Bronchitis is closely associated with asthma, as it involves the constriction of the airways in the lungs. Bacterial or viral infections can cause it, and if it reappears multiple times, it can become a chronic issue. A 2014 study from India found that bronchial asthma, a chronic form of the disease, was profoundly improved by the supplementation of curcumin. Thanks to a lack of "clinically significant adverse events," the scientists concluded that curcumin might be an effective add-on treatment for bronchitis and other bronchial dysfunction, without exposing patients to dangerous side effects.

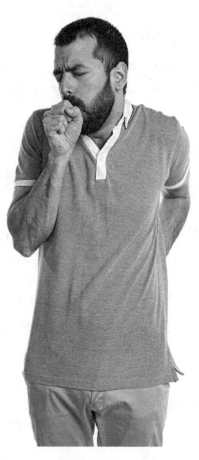

SKIN CONDITIONS

There are a number of skin conditions that turmeric may help prevent or treat. Since it has a wealth of antibacterial, anti-inflammatory and antifungal properties, many people claim that turmeric is great for preventing wrinkles and breakouts. It may also help to reduce the growth of skin tumors, according to a 2003 study, making it a nice salve for those concerned with contracting skin cancer. But turmeric may do more than just prevent cancer — as if that wasn't enough of a benefit. It many help treat psoriasis, eczema and wounds.

Soothes psoriasis

People who suffer from psoriasis experience thick, red, scaly lesions on the body. These unsightly lesions may even become infected if not treated properly. One of the causes of psoriasis is an elevation in PhK,

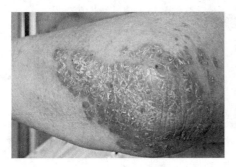

a protein produced by the body. In a study from the University of Texas MD Anderson Cancer Center, researchers investigated curcumin's ability to inhibit PhK. They found that it does, in fact, reduce the levels of PhK in psoriasis patients.

Another study, published in the *British Journal of Dermatology*, found that test subjects who did not receive treatment to lower PhK levels experienced the most significant psoriasis symptoms. However, subjects who were treated with curcumin — and who had been diagnosed with psoriasis — had the lowest PhK levels of the test groups, with the exception of the control subjects who had normal skin.

Supports skin healing

Turmeric may also help with wound healing. It has been shown to protect human skin cells from oxidative stress in laboratory experiments, indicating that it might be helpful in healing wounds as well. In addition, in a randomized, double-blind study published in *West Indian Medical Journal*, researchers found that women who had Caesarean operations benefited from using turmeric cream on their surgical wounds. Redness, swelling and bruising were all significantly reduced for test subjects who used the turmeric cream in contrast to those who did not.

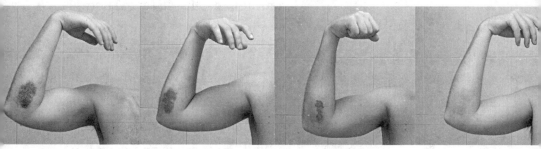

Treats eczema

Anyone who has had eczema knows the itchy red patches can drive you mad. But according to a review published in the *Journal of Medicinal Plants Research*, turmeric is one of four medicinal plants that can help with inflammation, itching, swelling, rashes or skin irritation.

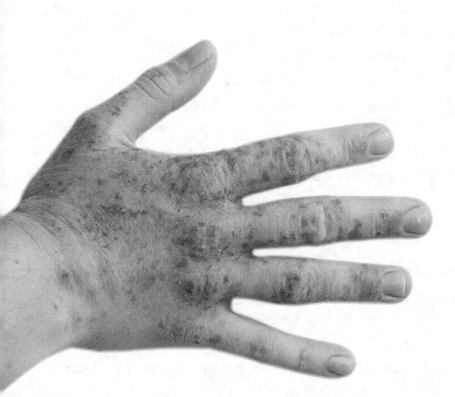

WEIGHT MANAGEMENT

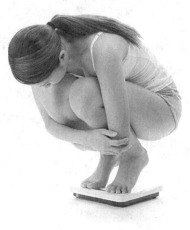

It appears that curcumin helps the body to metabolize fat, and it fights obesity. Here are some of the scientifically-backed conditions that turmeric may help in terms of weight management.

Lowers the accumulation of fat

Adding turmeric to your diet may help you lose weight. In a study conducted by Tohoku University Graduate School of Life Science and Agriculture in Sendai, Japan, curcuminoids — the compounds related to curcumin found in turmeric — were shown to prevent high-fat accumulation in rats. Researchers fed three groups of rats a high-fat diet. The control group received no curcumin, while another group received 0.2 grams, and the final group received a supplementation of 1 gram of curcumin.

The group of rats that received 1 gram of curcumin supplementation showed significantly lower triacylglycerol and cholesterol accumulation, lower rates of fat accumulation in the liver and lower body fat growth. The team concluded that curcumin alters the way fatty acid is metabolized in the body, and leads to lower cholesterol levels and body fat percentages.

Obesity and metabolic diseases

Metabolic abnormalities cause a number of health issues including cardiovascular disease, hypertension, type 2 diabetes and some cancers. Curcumin's anti-inflammatory properties have been shown to "interact with specific proteins in adipocytes, pancreatic cells, hepatic

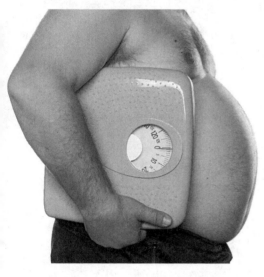

stellate cells, macrophages, and muscle cells, where it suppresses several cellular proteins," according to a 2011 Korean study. Turmeric's ability to pass through cell membranes and directly affect — and sometimes break down — proteins and fats mean it might be useful for combatting obesity and metabolic diseases.

Curcumin-free turmeric works too

As show here, a plethora of studies have focused on the benefits of curcumin, one of the primary compounds in turmeric. However, a 2013 study published in the journal *Molecular Nutrition & Food Research* found that curcumin-free turmeric also possesses anti-inflammatory, anti-cancer and anti-diabetic properties. So go ahead and add it to your favorite dishes, and don't forget to add some freshly ground black pepper to help your body access all of turmeric's benefits.

The Alternative Daily

RECIPES

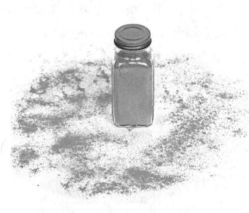

There's no limit to what you can do with turmeric, provided you have some recipes to guide you down the right path. The following section aims to do just that. We've provided 32 recipes involving turmeric and a mix of other potent ingredients to ensure you get the most out of this powerful spice. We've divided things up into three sections: health, beauty and just plain taste bud-tantalizing culinary concoctions!

Read on to find out how turmeric can literally, and metaphorically, spice up your life!

Turmeric recipes for health

Turmeric is fantastic for your health. The active ingredient curcumin, which gives turmeric its trademark color, is antiseptic, antibacterial, detoxifying, cancer-fighting, anti-inflammatory and anti-just-about-anything-else that's bad for your health. The following recipes are designed to nurture your health and have you feeling better than ever in no time.

Recipe #1: Hot Turmeric Coconut Drink

The coconut aspect to this tea might seem a little strange at first, but it adds a soothing richness to the drink that makes it that much more enjoyable to sip. Mix it up when you first feel a cold coming on, or simply drink it every day to keep your immune system tip top.

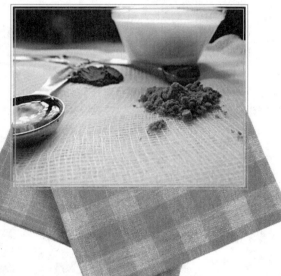

Ingredients

- 1 cup of full-fat coconut milk
- 1 tsp turmeric
- 1 tsp cinnamon
- 1 tsp raw honey or pure maple syrup
- 1/4 tsp cayenne pepper

Instructions

1. Pour the coconut milk into a pot and heat on the stove on low heat until hot, not boiling.
2. Add the rest of the ingredients, stirring with a spoon until smooth and combined.
3. Test the temperature, then drink straight away.

Recipe #2: Turmeric and Ginger Detox Blend

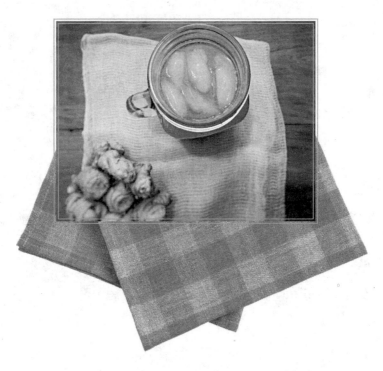

Ginger and turmeric are both well-researched detoxifiers. Throw in cayenne pepper, and you've got a powerful blend which flushes out harmful compounds from your body while reducing inflammation and alleviating pain. Yes, please!

Ingredients

- 2 inches of whole ginger root (or substitute 2 tsp ginger powder)
- 2 inches of whole turmeric root (or substitute 2 tsp turmeric powder)
- 1/2 tsp cayenne pepper
- Juice of 3 whole lemons
- 2 quarts of water

Equipment

- Juicer (optional)

Instructions

1. Use a juicer to extract the juice from your ginger root, turmeric root and lemons. If you don't have a juicer, use powdered ginger and turmeric, and simply cut your lemons in half and squeeze the juice out.
2. In a pitcher or large bowl, combine the juice (or powders) of ginger, turmeric and lemon with the water and cayenne pepper. Mix the ingredients thoroughly with a wooden spoon, adjusting ingredient ratios to suit your taste.
3. Allow to sit for 10 minutes to allow ingredient flavors and aromas to blend. Enjoy either at room temperature or over ice on a hot day.

Recipe #3: Turmeric Hot Toddy

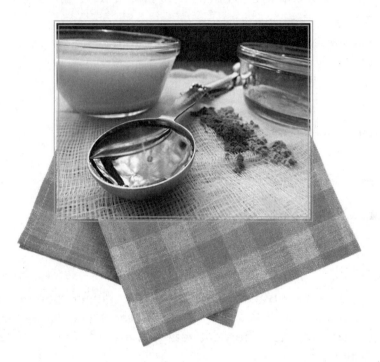

To your grandparents, or even your parents, a "hot toddy" was
something you were given when you were feeling a bit under the
weather or you just couldn't kick that cold. The generally held view
was "the stronger the better," and while we're not trying to get you
drunk, a healthy dash of whiskey goes a long way in this potent
concoction.

Ingredients

- 1 cup raw milk
- 1 tbsp raw honey
- 1 oz whiskey
- 1/4 tsp turmeric powder
- 1/4 tsp organic cinnamon powder

Instructions

1. Add the raw milk, honey and whiskey to a saucepan or pot and slowly warm on the stove until it starts to foam around the edges.
2. Pour into a mug, mix in the remaining ingredients with a teaspoon, and enjoy.

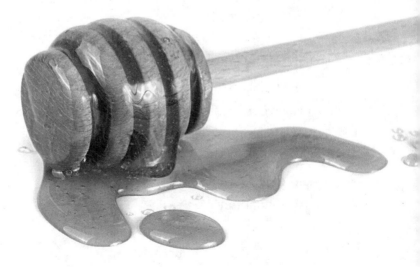

Recipe #4: Lemon and Ginger Refresher

Yes, another turmeric drink.
There's only so much liquid
your bladder can take,
right? But it's good to mix
up your health drinks on a
regular basis to ensure you
don't get tired of them. This
one has so many nurturing
ingredients we think you'll
agree that it's going to be a
regular, especially if you're
feeling less than ideal.

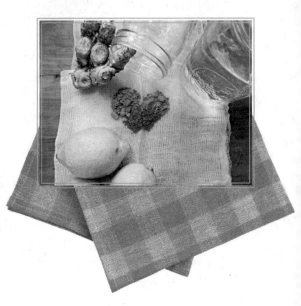

Ingredients

- 1 cup boiling water
- 1/2 tbsp turmeric powder
- 1 tbsp grated ginger root (or substitute 1/2 tbsp ginger powder)
- 1 handful cilantro, chopped fine
- 1 garlic clove, peeled and crushed
- 1 tbsp coconut oil
- Juice of 2 fresh lemons
- 5 whole peppercorns
- 1 tbsp raw honey

Instructions

1. Boil a generous cup of water on the stove or in a kettle, add to a teapot or tea strainer and pour in remaining ingredients.
2. Allow tea to steep for 10 to 15 minutes, strain and enjoy.

Recipe #5: Superfood Smoothie

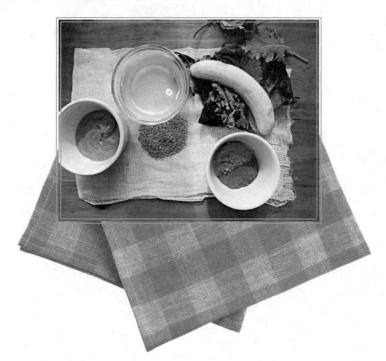

Short on time but need to get your morning nutrient fix? This smoothie is just the thing — it'll keep you satiated until lunch while boosting your immune system. It'll also provide your body with a powerful mix of nutrients to supercharge your energy levels.

Ingredients

- 1 cup roughly chopped organic kale (or collard greens)
- 1 chilled or frozen banana
- 1 cup pure coconut water
- 2 tbsp almond butter
- 1 tbsp flax oil (or 2 tbsp flaxseeds)
- 1/2 tsp cinnamon powder
- 1 tsp turmeric powder

Equipment

- Blender

Instructions

1. Place all the ingredients into a blender and churn it up until smooth. If necessary, use a wooden spoon to scoop the bits of leaves back into the general mix, then re-blend to ensure you get all the good stuff.
2. Drink immediately, or store covered in the fridge overnight for a morning meal on-the-go!

Recipe #6: Rejuvenating Turmeric Juice

Need a break from all these health smoothies and teas? How about a delicious rejuvenating turmeric juice? To avoid making a complete mess of the kitchen, you'll need a juicer for this one.

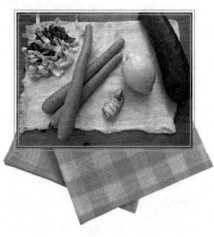

Ingredients

- 2 inches of whole turmeric root
- 1 cup organic romaine lettuce
- 3 organic carrots
- 1 organic English cucumber (if another type of cucumber, peel the skin first)
- 1 lemon with skin removed

Equipment

- Juicer

Instructions

1. Thoroughly wash all the ingredients and set aside.
2. Juice each ingredient in the following order: turmeric, romaine lettuce, carrots, lemon and cucumber. If necessary, add water to ensure good consistency for drinking.
3. Stir mixture and drink immediately.

The Alternative Daily

Recipe #7: Turmeric Anti-Cancer Spice

This recipe is a simple one but a vitally important one. Research indicates that adding turmeric to meat which has been cooked at high heat, such as on the grill or pan frying, can reduce its heterocyclic amine (HCA) level by 40 percent. HCAs have been strongly associated with development of various types of cancer, so reducing the HCA content of your meat is a big deal.

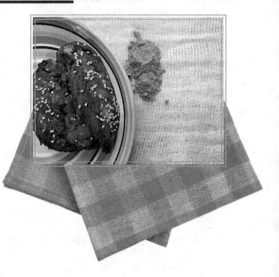

Ingredients

- Organic turmeric powder (or substitute freshly grated organic turmeric root)

Instructions

1. After you've cooked your beef, chicken, fish or other type of meat over high heat (pan frying, barbecuing, grilling, etc.) simply spring a healthy dose of turmeric powder onto your meat and rub it in with some salt and pepper. Not only will this give your meat a delicious exotic flavor, it will dramatically reduce the carcinogenicity of your meat. You're welcome!

Recipe #8: Homemade Curry Powder Blend

These days, you never know what's in the products you buy. If you happen to take a look at the back of the packaging for some of the spices you've been buying for a long time, you might be shocked to see that many have hydrogenated oils added to them. Yuck! Why not take control and concoct your own delicious, anti-inflammatory, nutrient-dense spice mix?

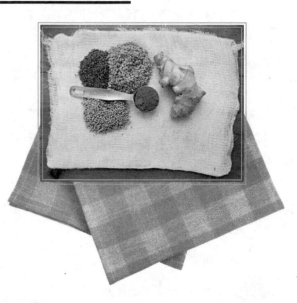

Ingredients

- 3 inches of whole turmeric root
- 2 tbsp whole cumin seeds, toasted
- 2 tbsp whole coriander seeds, toasted
- 1 tbsp wholegrain mustard seeds
- 1 tsp cayenne pepper powder

Equipment

- Blender

The Alternative Daily

Instructions

1. Place the turmeric root into a good blender (i.e. a Vitamix) and blend until the root becomes ground up as much as possible.

2. Place the turmeric on a baking sheet, spread out thinly, and put in the oven on 200°F for around 2 hours, or until it has dried out sufficiently. If you're feeling lazy, you can just go out and buy some pure organic turmeric powder and skip this step!

3. Throw all the ingredients into a glass container with an airtight lid.

4. Shake well to combine.

5. Store in a cool dry place. When ready to use, place in a grinder and sprinkle generously over the dish of your choice!

Recipe #9: Golden Milk

It sounds kind of mystical, and perhaps it is! Golden milk is an ancient Ayurvedic concoction that provides your body with a potent mix of vital mix of fats, nutrients and anti-inflammatories. Plus, it tastes delicious, particularly on a cold winter night or instead of your plain old warm milk before bed.

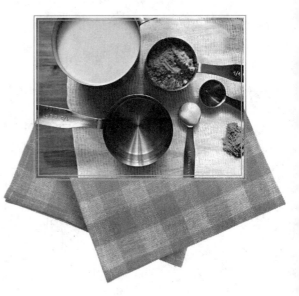

Ingredients

- 1/2 cup filtered or spring water
- 1/4 cup ground turmeric
- 1 cup raw milk
- 1/2 tsp coconut oil (or grass-fed ghee)
- 1/2 tsp ground cinnamon
- 1 tsp raw honey

Instructions

1. Bring the water to a low simmer on the stove.
2. Mix in the turmeric and stir constantly until a thick paste forms.
3. Warm the raw milk with 1/2 tsp of the turmeric paste on the stove, stirring occasionally.
4. After 5 minutes, mix in the coconut oil or whee. Also add the ground cinnamon and raw honey to taste.
5. Drink immediately, and store the remaining turmeric paste in the fridge for up to 2 weeks.

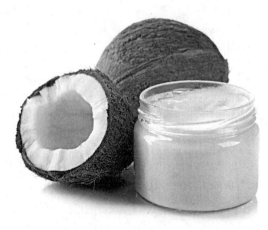

Recipe #10: Golden Honey

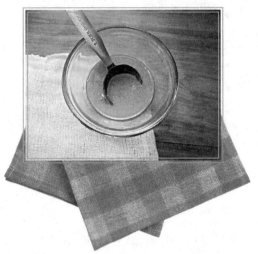

While we're on the topic of golden things, it seems like a good time to introduce another of turmeric's great talents: fighting colds. This simple mixture, so named on account of the fact that turmeric makes almost everything it touches a golden color, helps to boost your immune system, fight inflammation and soothe a sore throat all in one fell swoop. Plus it has honey in it, so there'll be no complaining from your family if you make them take a dollop of it when they're sick.

Ingredients

- 1 tbsp organic turmeric powder
- 7 tbsp raw honey

Instructions

1. In a glass jar or stainless steel mixing bowl, mix together ground turmeric with raw honey. Whenever you feel a cold or sore throat coming on, spoon out a generous dollop and swallow it.

It's important that you use only raw honey. Pasteurized honey doesn't have the active enzymes which fight bacteria in your throat and help you digest the sugars and nutrients in the honey more efficiently.

Recipe #11: Turmeric and Chia Smoothie

This smoothie combines the detoxifying, anti-inflammatory, hormone-balancing benefits of turmeric with the cleansing power of chia seeds and the digestion-boosting powers of pineapple to give you a drink of epic proportions. Use your newfound health power wisely.

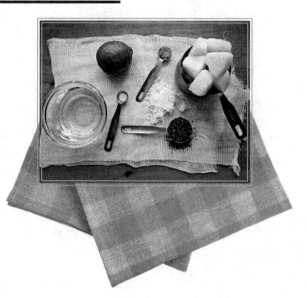

Ingredients

- 1 cup chopped frozen pineapple
- 1/2 tsp turmeric powder (or 1-inch whole turmeric root)
- 1 tbsp chia seeds
- 1 tbsp shredded coconut
- 1 lime with skin removed
- 1 cup filtered water
- Pinch of Himalayan pink salt

Equipment

- Blender

Instructions

1. Add all the ingredients to your blender and blend on high until smooth and well combined.
2. Pour into a glass and enjoy!

Recipe #12: Homemade Mustard

We all know the amazing health benefits that turmeric possesses by now, and wholegrain mustard seeds are a cancer-fighting, anti-inflammatory, thyroid-boosting, nutritional powerhouse. Combine the two, and you've got yourself a delicious, nutritious, disease-preventing homemade mustard to add to many of your meaty dishes and cheese platters.

Ingredients

- 1/2 cup wholegrain mustard seeds
- 2 tbsp white wine vinegar
- 1 tbsp water
- 1 tsp turmeric powder
- 1 tsp salt

Instructions

1. Combine all the ingredients in a glass jar and mix together with a spoon.
2. Seal the jar securely with a lid and store in the fridge.

Recipe #13: Turmeric Pickle

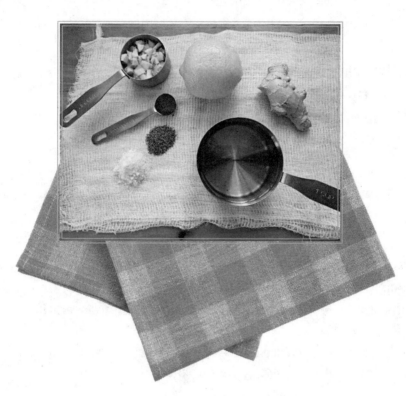

Everyone needs at least one jar of delicious pickles sitting in their fridge, ready to add moisture and tang to a dry sandwich or as a healthy condiment to a meaty dish. Why not combine the versatility and flavor of your average pickle with the health-giving powers of turmeric, in wonderful symbiosis with ginger and cardamom.

Ingredients

- 1/4 cup fresh organic ginger root, diced
- 1/4 cup fresh organic turmeric root, diced
- 1 cup avocado oil
- 1 tsp black mustard seeds
- 1/2 tsp chili powder
- 2 tsp Himalayan pink salt
- Juice of 1 whole lemon

Instructions

1. Roughly dice the organic ginger and turmeric without removing the skin.
2. Heat some of the avocado oil in a pan and add all the spices other than the ginger and turmeric.
3. Take the pan off the heat as soon as the mustard seeds start to pop.
4. Add the spice mixture to the diced ginger and turmeric in a glass jar, along with the rest of the oil, salt and lemon juice.
5. Seal the jar with a good airtight lid.

Your delicious pickle mixture won't get funky in your fridge for around 2 to 3 months, and we suspect you'll eat it all well before then.

Recipe #14: Anti-Hangover Turmeric Milk

We've all had those nights where that
wine or beer just goes down way
too smoothly, resulting in a morning
where your head is pounding and
your body seems hell-bent on making
you pay for your discrepancies the
night before. If this is you, try the
following recipe — it might just make
your hungover morning a whole lot
more enjoyable.

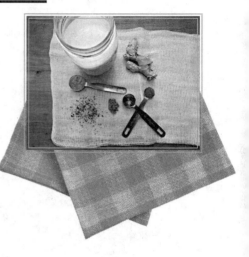

Ingredients

- 2 cups raw grass-fed milk
- 1 tsp turmeric powder
- 3 whole black peppercorns
- 1/8 tsp ground cardamom
- 1/2 ginger root, roughly chopped
- 1/4 tsp cinnamon
- 1/2 tsp raw honey

Instructions

1. Add all the ingredients to a pot and heat on low until they're
   mixed together and just starting to froth (shouldn't be too hot to
   touch).
2. Remove immediately from heat and enjoy.

The Alternative Daily

Recipe #15: Turmeric, Watermelon and Pineapple Smoothie

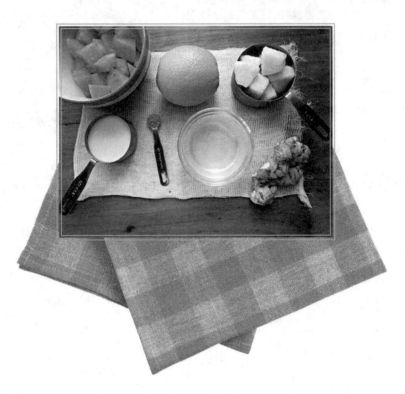

This recipe combines the nutritional might of four fantastic natural foods: turmeric, watermelon, pineapple and coconut. The result is a smoothie which tastes delicious, and it's so healthy it'll heal you from the inside out.

Ingredients

- 2 cups frozen watermelon, cut into rough chunks
- 1 cup frozen pineapple, cut into rough chunks
- 1 peeled orange, seeds removed if possible
- 1/2 cup coconut milk
- 1 1/2 cups coconut water
- 1 tsp grated fresh ginger
- 1/2 tsp turmeric powder

Equipment

- Blender

Instructions

1. Throw all the ingredients into a high speed blender and blend until smooth.
2. Use a large spoon to place the mixture into serving glasses, and enjoy!

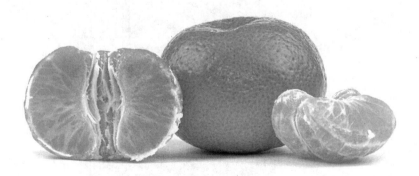

TURMERIC RECIPES FOR BEAUTY

As with many things in life, what's good for our insides is also good for our outsides. Turmeric is no exception. In fact, turmeric is a shining example of how food which nurtures our health also amplifies and improves our beauty. It can be used as an effective natural replacement for many skin, hair and even nail products. It provides a non-toxic cheap alternative to those nasty conventional cosmetics and beauty products on supermarket and drugstore shelves. Throw all your beauty products out! There's a new kid in town, and it goes by the name of turmeric!

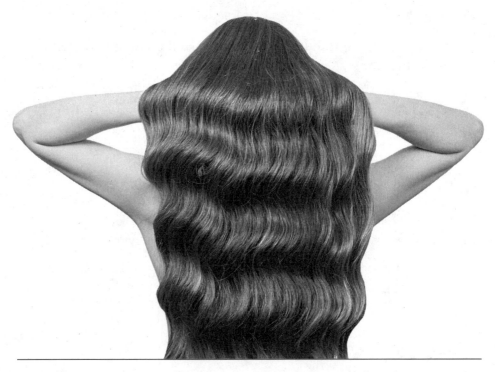

Recipe #16: Anti-Acne Turmeric Face Mask

Despite all the fancy treatments and creams you've tried over the years, your battle with acne rages on. Maybe it's time to take a step back and turn to simple, wholesome ingredients to solve your pimple problem.

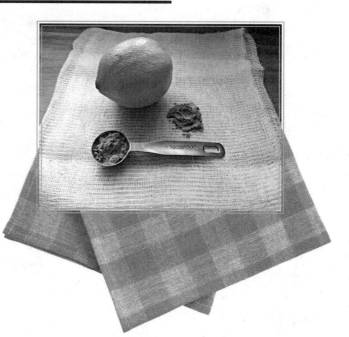

Ingredients

- 1 tsp turmeric powder
- 1 tsp sandalwood powder
- Juice from half a lemon

Instructions

1. In a small glass or stainless steel bowl, use a spoon to mix together the turmeric, sandalwood, and lemon juice.
2. Apply the mixture to your face and leave it on for 10 minutes.
3. Rinse off with warm water. Simple as that.

The Alternative Daily

Recipe #17: Turmeric Mask For Youthful Skin

The antioxidants overflowing from a simple jar of turmeric make it an excellent choice for concocting highly effective homemade anti-aging products. This recipe is easy to put together and can be made with any of your favorite beneficial oils.

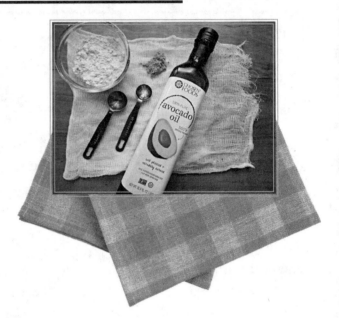

Ingredients

- 1 1/2 tbsp turmeric powder
- 1/2 cup garbanzo (or chickpea) flour
- 1/2 tsp avocado oil (or hemp seed, almond, extra virgin olive)
- 1 to 2 tsp filtered water

Instructions

1. Mix together the turmeric powder and chickpea flour and set aside in an airtight container until you are ready to make your skin mask.

2. To make the skin mask, mix 1 tablespoon of the flour mixture with 1/2 teaspoon of your oil of choice, adding just enough water to make a thick paste.

3. Gently rub the paste onto your face, neck and any areas which are looking in need of attention. Avoid getting it too close to your eyes, and keep it well away from your clothes!

4. Leave the mask on for 15 to 20 minutes, then wash it off with warm water in the shower.

Recipe #18: Turmeric Eye Stye Treatment

If you suspect you're in the process of developing a nasty pocket of inflammation around your eye — called a stye — we have just the thing. It combines the anti-inflammatory powers of turmeric with the probiotic power of kefir to provide one serious stye-destroying paste.

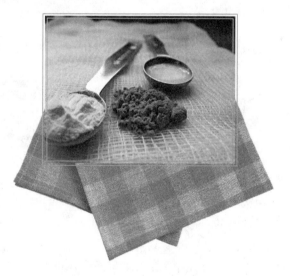

Ingredients

- 1/4 tsp turmeric powder
- 1/4 tsp arrowroot powder
- 1/2 tsp raw milk or coconut milk kefir

Instructions

1. In a small bowl, use a thin utensil like a chopstick or the handle of a spoon to mix together the ingredients.
2. Add one drop of tap or filtered water at a time until the mix becomes a thick paste.
3. Carefully apply to the affected area with a clean finger, and allow to dry.
4. Leave on until the swelling in your eye reduces or goes away completely.
5. Carefully rinse off with your eye closed.

Recipe #19: Anti-Oil Turmeric Face Mask

Turmeric is excellent for skin which is excessively oily, as it helps to regulate the production of sebum, an oily substance produced by your skin's sebaceous glands. Combine it with a few other useful natural ingredients, and you've got yourself an effective anti-oil facial mask.

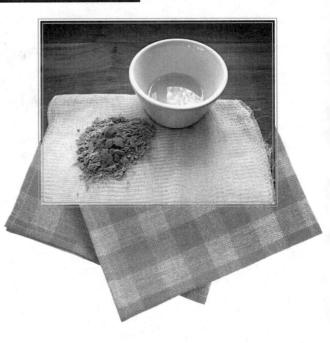

Ingredients

- 1/2 tsp turmeric powder
- 1 1/2 tbsp sandalwood powder
- 3 tbsp pure orange juice

Instructions

1. Mix all the ingredients together in a bowl to make a rough paste.
2. Rub the mixture gently into your face, using circular motions.
3. Leave on for 15 minutes to allow time to soak into your pores
4. Rinse off with warm water.

Recipe #20: Turmeric Stretch Mark Treatment

Whether from historic struggles with weight, or the aftermath of childbirth, many of us have come to accept the fact that stretch marks are here to stay. That doesn't have to be the case, and in fact these marks can be diminished or even banished completely with a very simple natural daily treatment involving turmeric, gram flour and yogurt or raw milk.

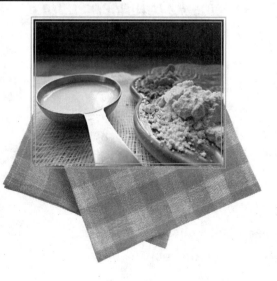

Ingredients

- 1/2 tsp turmeric powder
- 1 tsp gram chickpea flour (or garbanzo flour)
- 1 tbsp yogurt (or raw milk)

Instructions

1. In a bowl, mix together the turmeric and gram flour.
2. Add the raw milk or yogurt slowly until it forms a thick paste.
3. Rub the paste onto your stretch marks.
4. Leave on for around 20 minutes, then rinse off. Apply as many as three times daily for as long as necessary.

Recipe #21: Turmeric Burn Relief

Burns are nasty, and left untreated can become infected and quickly make your life very unenjoyable. This recipe utilizes the anti-inflammatory abilities of turmeric and the cooling, hydrating effects of aloe vera to minimize pain from a burn and ensure it heals quickly.

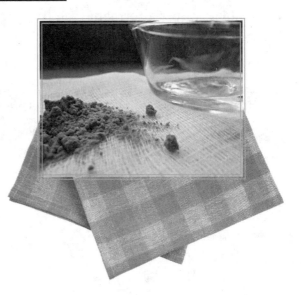

Ingredients

- 1 tsp turmeric powder
- 2 tsp pure aloe vera gel

Instructions

1. Mix the two ingredients together to form a thick paste.
2. Gently apply to the burn area.
3. Leave on for 30 minutes to an hour, rinse off with cool water, and apply again if necessary.

Recipe #22: Turmeric Facial Hair Remover

Applying this natural recipe to your face on a daily basis for about a month can help to inhibit facial hair growth and ensure you don't need to keep using those unpleasant facial waxing kits or other uncomfortable means. It asks for Kasturi Manjal turmeric, the wild counterpart to the usual cooking turmeric. If you can't find any of this exotic-sounding spice in your local health food store, using the conventional turmeric powder should also be okay.

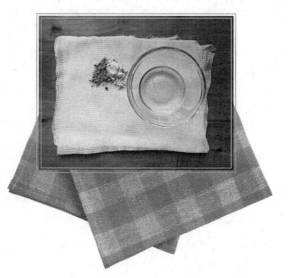

Ingredients

- 1 tsp kasturi turmeric powder
- 1 tsp gram chickpea flour (or garbanzo flour)
- 1 1/2 tsp filtered water

Instructions

1. Mix together the turmeric and gram flour.
2. Slowly add a few drops of the filtered water, one at a time, until the mixture resembles a thick paste.
3. Rub the paste onto areas of your face prone to excessive facial hair growth on a daily basis, leaving on for 15 to 20 minutes, then rinsing off with warm water.

Recipe #23: Turmeric Night Cream

Our body does most of its growth and healing while we slumber, so what better time to rejuvenate and enliven your skin as well? This natural night cream does just that, helping to provide your skin with the nutrients and compounds it needs to stay young and firm, all while you peacefully snore away the hours.

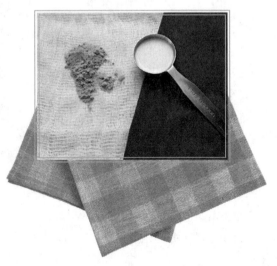

Ingredients

- 2 tsp turmeric powder
- 1 tbsp raw milk or plain full-fat yogurt

Instructions

1. In a glass jar, mix together the turmeric powder and raw milk. Depending on how watery the mixture is, add more turmeric powder to thicken the mixture or more milk or yogurt to water it down. You want the night cream to be thick enough that it doesn't run down your face when you apply it.

2. Rub the mixture onto your face just before bed, put a towel on your pillow to ensure that you don't stain anything, and let yourself drift away with the knowledge that your face will be that much more youthful in the morning.

3. Rinse the cream off in the shower in the morning. Try to do this routine around twice a week for more youthful, vibrant skin.

Recipe #24: Turmeric Foot Cream

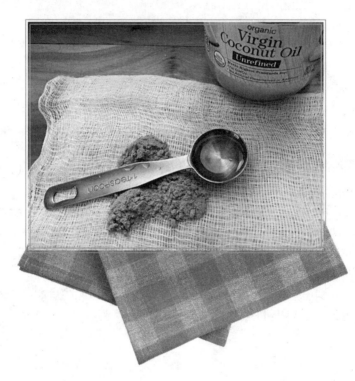

While we're on the subject of creams, it's about time you started giving your feet a little more TLC by putting some cream on them every now and then. When neglected, our feet can become dry, cracked and develop sores. They can host a range of different conditions which make every day a whole lot harder. Try this natural foot cream to treat dry, cracked feet and keep them nice and supple. They'll thank you for it!

Ingredients

- 3 tsp turmeric powder
- 1 tsp coconut oil (or castor oil)

Instructions

1. Make a paste by combining turmeric powder with coconut oil above room temperature (i.e., in its liquid form) or castor oil. If the paste is too dry, add more oil as necessary.
2. Using strong circular motions, use your hands to massage the paste onto the bottom of your feet, paying particular attention to the heels.
3. Sit back, put your feet up, and leave the foot cream on for 15 minutes before rinsing off with warm water.

To increase the effectiveness of the cream, try having a warm bath immediately after removing the foot cream. After the bath, rub some coconut or castor oil on your feet to lock in the moisture, and your feet will feel like new!

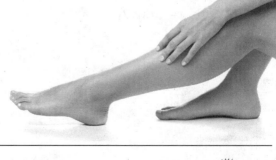

Recipe #25: Egg Yolk Moisturizing Mask

This natural face mask works wonders on dry skin. The egg yolk promotes skin repair and provides a range of B vitamins. The olive oil hydrates your skin and locks in the moisture. The turmeric gives your skin a vibrant, healthy glow.

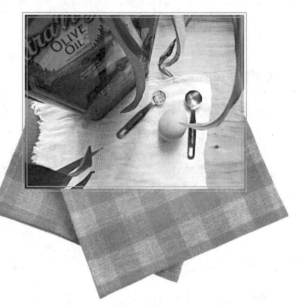

Ingredients

- 1 free-range egg yolk
- 1/2 tsp turmeric powder
- 1 tsp extra virgin olive oil

Instructions

1. Use a fork or whisk to scramble the egg yolk in a small bowl.
2. Mix in the turmeric and olive oil to make a paste.
3. Apply the mixture to your face, let it dry for 20 minutes, and rinse off with warm water.

Recipe #26: DIY Turmeric Face Mask

This do-it-yourself face mask provides your skin with a potent blend of antioxidants. It encourages cell repair, reduces cell damage, exfoliates your skin, improves texture, fights inflammatory skin conditions like eczema, psoriasis and acne, and evens out skin tone. Oh, did we mention that it reduces wrinkles? Yup, it does that, too.

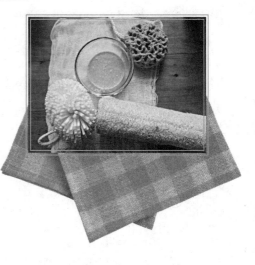

Ingredients

- 2 tbsp rice flour or gram (chickpea) flour
- 1 tsp turmeric powder
- 3 tbsp raw milk (or plain yogurt)
- 1/2 tsp raw honey

Instructions

1. Mix the flour, turmeric, milk and honey together to make a paste.
2. Apply a thin layer of the mixture to your face to form a mask, and let it dry over approximately 20 minutes.
3. Rinse off in the shower with warm water, rubbing gently to remove.
4. After the shower, rub a small amount of coconut oil on your face to seal in the moisture.

Recipe #27: Turmeric Skin Exfoliator

Over time, dead skin cells can build up and begin to clog our pores and contribute to a range of skin conditions. One of the best ways to remove dead skin cells and keep your skin looking young and fresh is to exfoliate — and we have just the thing.

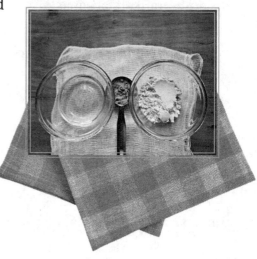

Ingredients

- 2 tbsp gram (chickpea) flour
- 1 tbsp turmeric powder
- 3 tbsp filtered water

Instructions

1. In a small bowl, mix together the gram flour and turmeric powder.
2. Gradually add water until the mixture forms a thick, gritty paste.
3. Use your hands or a sponge to firmly scrub your skin with the paste while taking a warm bath or shower, then rinse off.

Doing this on a regular basis can keep your skin clear and nurtured-looking, and help prevent the development of various unsightly skin conditions.

TURMERIC RECIPES FOR YOUR TASTEBUDS

It's all very well whipping together magical tonics, nutrient-dense smoothies or skin-bedazzling concoctions, but sometimes you just want to take a break from the whole beauty and health scene. We get it. So, with you in mind, we've put together a series of food recipes which ensure you get the same health-promoting benefits of turmeric while also feeding yourself and your family. And your tastebuds won't complain, either.

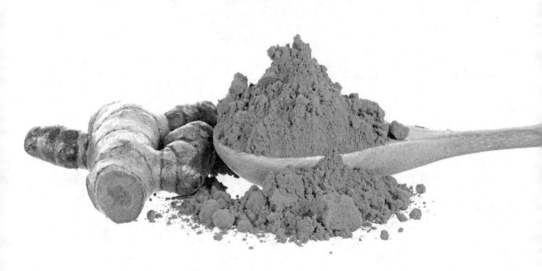

Recipe #28: Sprouted Lentil Burger

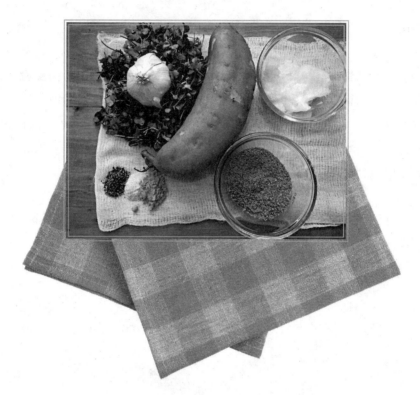

If you're taking a break from meat or vegetarianism is your thing, this burger is right up your alley. It provides an excellent meatless source of protein. Plus, the sprouted lentils provide a wide range of vitamins and enzymes, and it tastes mighty fine as well.

Ingredients

- 2 cups sprouted lentils
- 1 boiled sweet potato, mashed
- 2 tbsp grass-fed butter or coconut oil
- 3 tbsp ground flaxseed
- 2 cloves garlic
- 1 tsp Himalayan pink salt
- 1 tsp pepper
- 1 tsp turmeric powder

Equipment

- Food processor (or large blender)

Instructions

1. Steam or boil the sweet potato, then remove the skin and mash.
2. In a food processor or large blender, combine all the ingredients until well mixed.
3. With your hands, form the mixture into patties.
4. Cook in a skillet with the butter or coconut oil on medium heat. When the bottom of the patties begin to brown, flip and cook the other side for a few minutes.
5. Serve with a side salad, perhaps a little cheese and your favorite condiments. The turmeric pickle recipe (#13) would pair with the patties rather nicely!

Recipe #29: Turmeric Eggs

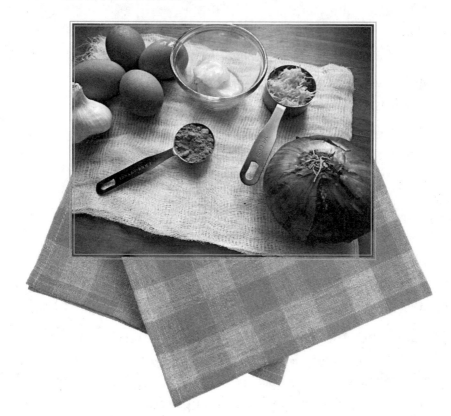

Eggs are a nutritional powerhouse, particularly if they're from organic-fed, free-range hens. But if you have them on a regular basis, they can become a little boring. Why not spice things up a little with this delicious recipe? It employs the amazing earthy taste of turmeric and throws in a few extra tasty ingredients to ensure your tastebuds are not left wanting. Your biggest problem will be trying to stop eating them!

Ingredients

- 4 large free-range eggs
- 2 tbsp ghee
- 1/2 cup of chopped red onion
- 3 cloves garlic, chopped
- 1 tbsp turmeric
- 1/4 cup grated cheese

Instructions

1. In a skillet or cast iron frying pan, sauté the onion and garlic in the ghee on medium heat for around 10 minutes.
2. After the vegetables have softened, add in the cheese, eggs and turmeric. Continue to cook the mixture for another 5 to 10 minutes, stirring constantly.
3. Once the mixture has cooled sufficiently, serve and enjoy!

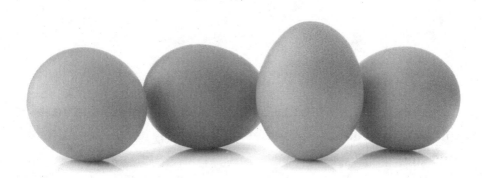

Recipe #30: Turmeric Carrot Soup

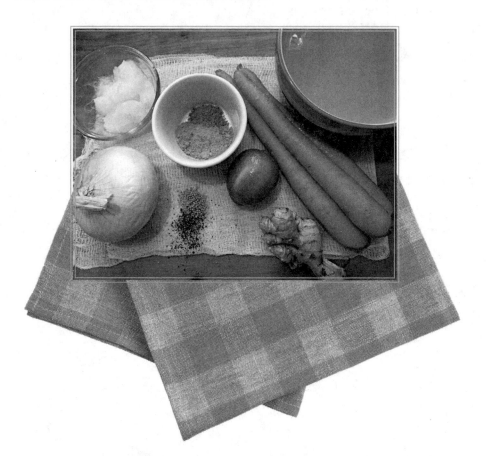

Carrots are great for your health and taste amazing when they're cooked the right way. Combine them with the earthy deliciousness of turmeric and you've got yourself an amazingly nutritious, finger-licking good soup!

Ingredients

- 4 tbsp coconut oil
- 6 cups chicken broth
- 5 cups carrots, thinly sliced
- 2 cups chopped onion
- 2 tsp turmeric
- 1 tbsp fresh ginger, minced
- 1 tsp coriander seeds
- 3/4 tsp mustard seeds
- 3 tsp fresh lime juice
- Himalayan pink salt to taste
- Pepper to taste

Equipment

- Blender

Instructions

1. Melt the coconut oil in a soup pot over medium heat.
2. Add the coriander seeds, mustard seeds, turmeric and ginger. Stir for a minute, then add some salt and pepper.
3. Add the onions and sauté till soft and clear.
4. Add the chicken broth and carrots, reduce to low heat and cook for around 30 minutes.
5. Remove from heat, pour the soup into a blender and puree until smooth.

6. Return the pureed mixture to the pot, stir in the lime juice and add more salt and pepper to taste.

7. Serve with an optional garnish of raw yogurt or raw sour cream and parsley.

Recipe #31: Chicken Tikka Masala

What kind of people would we be if we didn't throw in a classic Indian curry recipe, done the healthy way? We've turned what can be a long, complicated dish into a quick, easy one, and of course... properties were valid turmeric plays a starring role!

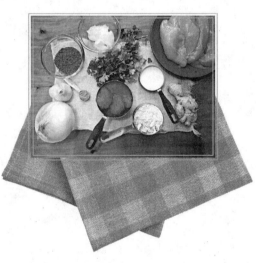

Ingredients

- 4 tsp garam masala
- 1/2 tsp Himalayan pink salt
- 1/2 tsp turmeric
- 1/2 cup rice flour
- 1 lb chicken tenders
- 4 tsp coconut oil
- 6 cloves garlic, minced
- 1 large chopped onion
- 4 tsp minced ginger root

- 1 cup plum tomatoes
- 1/3 cup whipping cream
- 1/2 cup chopped fresh cilantro

Instructions

1. In a bowl, mix together the garam masala, salt and turmeric.
2. Spread out the rice flour on a plate, sprinkle over a 1/2 tsp of the garam masala mixture, and roll the chicken in the flour and spice.
3. Heat 2 tsp of coconut oil in a large skillet over medium-high heat. Cook the chicken until brown, around 2 minutes per side. Set aside.
4. Heat the remaining 2 tsp of coconut oil in another pan over medium to low heat. Add the garlic, onion and ginger and cook for around 5 minutes, stirring constantly.
5. Add the remaining garam masala and stir for 1 minute.
6. Sprinkle the remaining rice flour left over from the chicken coating and stir until coated.
7. Add the tomatoes, bring mixture to a simmer, and stir for another 5 minutes.
8. Stir in the cream and add the chicken to the mixture. Bring to a simmer again and cook over low heat until the chicken is cooked through, approximately 5 minutes.
9. Garnish with cilantro, and let your tastebuds have their way!

CONCLUSION

Well, if you weren't crazy about turmeric before, you probably are now! Turmeric is such a versatile spice, and it's just so darn good for you. There's no reason not to use it every single day. We hope you enjoy using turmeric for your health, your beauty and your tastebuds as much as we do!